FINGER ACUPRESSURE*

(Revised/Enlarged Edition)

By Pedro Chan

*FINGER ACUPUNCTURE

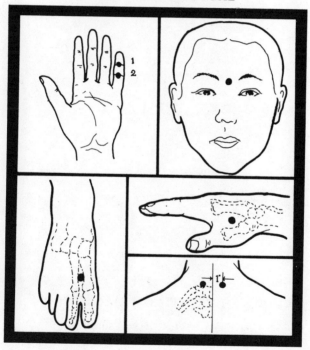

TREATMENT FOR MANY COMMON AILMENTS
FROM MIGRAINE TO INSOMNIA
BY USING FINGER MASSAGE ON ACUPUNCTURE POINTS

PRICE/STERN/SLOAN
Publishers, Inc., Los Angeles
1980

SIXTH PRINTING – MAY, 1980

Copyright© 1974, 1975 by Pedro Chan
Published by Price/Stern/Sloan Publishers, Inc.
410 North La Cienega Boulevard, Los Angeles, California 90048

ISBN: 0-8431-0344-2
Library of Congress Catalog Card No.: 74-76761

NOTE

Finger acupuncture is never a cure. It is also not the intention of the author to provide a substitute for acupuncture or conventional therapy. Finger acupuncture should be used only as a supplement. By all means, see a licensed acupuncturist or physician for any condition requiring medical treatment.

CONTENTS

FOREWORD

Acupuncture is an ancient Chinese art of healing by inserting fine needles in the body at certain well-defined points. The idea that a fine needle pricking the skin at the back of the knee (Wei-chung, Bladder 54) can in a few minutes relieve a long-standing low-back pain; that one painlessly pierced at a point on the back of the hand near the base of the thumb (Ho-ku, Large intestine 4) can relieve toothache or even induce anesthesia for tonsillectomy; or that one placed in the skin about three inches below the kneecap just outside the tibia (Tsu-san-li, Stomach 36) can relieve stomachache, cure gastritis, combat general fatigue and, at the same time, conserve robust health, may sound fantastic to the Western mind. Nonetheless, the experience of those knowledgeable in acupuncture either as a doctor, patient, or objective observer seems to confirm some, at least, of these claims.

There are some 500-800 acupuncture points or spots as shown by various Chinese and Japanese charts. Exactly 669 points are listed in Dr. Chu Lien's *Hsin Chen Chiu Hsueh* (Modern Acupuncture), a standard textbook on acupuncture used in present-day China. Many new points have been discovered in China in recent years. There is definitely some relation and connection between point(s) of skin and disorder(s) of the human body. The question is to get them stimulated. There are quite a number of ways of stimulation, such as needles, moxa, electricity, injection or even finger pressure.

During my recent trip to China, I witnessed treatments using finger pressure for relieving toothache or tooth extraction. The method is simple, easy, and causes no pain to the patient. Mr. Chan, an associate of mine in Chinese medicine, has used his experience, and others', to illustrate with simplicity, the essence of finger acupuncture. This appears to be the first guide book of such a technique in the English language, and should be a good guide for those beginners without previous knowledge of acupuncture.

James Y. P. Chen, M.D.
Vice President of
American Society of Chinese Medicine
President, Acupuncture Research Institute

INTRODUCTION

Acupuncture is the art of healing involving the insertion of needles into some specific points of the body. These points are called acupuncture points. Finger acupuncture, as the name implies, is that kind of healing which involves finger massage over the acupuncture points. The author, using his own experience, as well as other professionals, has picked out the most effective acupuncture points to treat certain common disorders, by utilizing the finger technique. It is simple, easy harmless, and effective in most cases. It can be used anywhere and by anyone without special knowledge. Subjects will not be scared because there is no needle insertion. And in practical use, this treatment can be applied as a first-aid measure because of its efficacy and convenience. Also, no equipment or drug is needed in the procedure.

However, finger acupuncture is never a cure. It is also not the intention of the author to provide a substitute for acupuncture or conventional therapy. Finger acupuncture should only be used as a supplement. By all means, see a licensed acupuncturist or physician for any condition requiring medical treatment.

Pedro Chan
Los Angeles, California
March, 1974

In response to the many letters and inquiries I received from readers of the first two editions of *Finger Acupressure*, I have added 21 new pages. This revised, enlarged edition covers 10 additional ailments, including the common cold. I hope they will be of additional help to old as well as new readers.

Pedro Chan
Los Angeles, California
January, 1975

THE ESSENTIALS OF FINGER ACUPUNCTURE

Posture

No matter what the posture is — lying down or sitting up — the subject must be relaxed, comfortable and natural, and the practitioner must be able to fully utilize his finger movement and strength.

Finger Pressure

It varies with the physique of the subject. Generally, light pressure is applied on subjects in the following categories:
1) 1st time subject.
2) Acute pain.
3) Swelling.
4) With weak, or loose muscles.
5) With complications such as high blood pressure, Addisonian anemia, or heart trouble.

Hard pressure is applied on the following subjects:
1) Chronic problem.
2) Without other complications.
3) Not overly-tired.

Manipulation

Press against the point of the skin surface, in a small circular movement, about 2 or 3 cycles per second. Points are always applied bilaterally. Start with one point at a time and when you master this technique, you may work bilaterally and simultaneously with your two hands.

Period of Treatment

It can range from one minute to five minutes for each point per treatment, once a day, or whenever you have the problem, or whenever you feel you wish to do it.

Caution

Please keep the following in mind.

1) Keep the treatment room warm, but well ventilated. This will help the subject to be comfortable, and prevent him from becoming chilled.

2) The practitioner should keep his hands clean and warm, and his nails trimmed to prevent injuring the subject or making him nervous and tense.

3) Never work on a subject if he has a full stomach.

4) The treatment is not to be applied on pregnant women, or serious cardiac patients.

5) Avoid working on skin surface of contusion, scar or infection.

6) Stop treatment if the symptom is being aggravated, and no relief is observed.

Forbidden Diet

Diet plays an important role in Chinese medicine, as some foods have certain counter or irritating effects on the patient. It is wise, therefore, to avoid the following foods during the treatment:

1) Iced food or drink.

2) Sour foods, such as vinegar, pickle, lemon, pineapple....

3) Alcoholic drinks.

4) Irritating food such as pepper, hot sauce, spices.....

5) Seafood with shell such as lobster, shrimp, crab.....

Please Note:

For some ailments, it is necessary to use pressure on more than one acupuncture point. In this case, when more than one is shown, use in the sequence pictured.

ALPHABETICAL LIST OF DISORDERS

Simplicity is the main feature of this book.

Following each disorder is the name of the point and its description of the location. It is again illustrated by:

1) Drawing an anatomical location, with relation to skeletal structure. And

2) Picture showing live treatment.

Follow the instruction to locate the correct point. Press firmly and deeply. In doing this correctly, the subject should feel some sensation of numbness, soreness, swelling and heaviness.

Point	Location & Technique
Tsu-san-li	About 3 inches below the kneecap, 1 inch lateral to the tibia. Lie or sit down. Use thumb to press down, then massage upward.

足
三
里

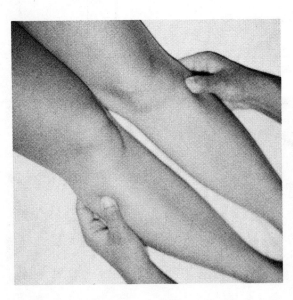

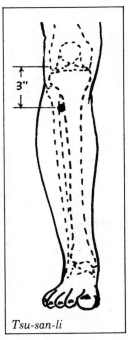

Tsu-san-li

Point

Chung-wan

Location & Technique

About 4 inches above the navel, along the midline of the abdominal surface.

Lie or sit down.

Use thumb or palm to massage inward.

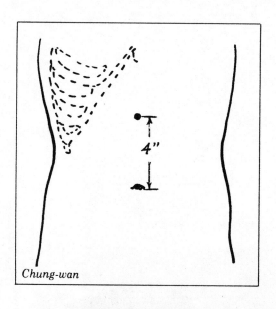

4"

Chung-wan

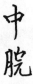

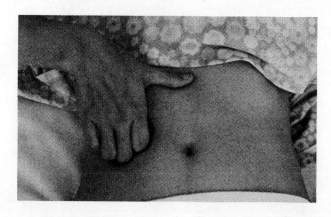

Point	Location & Technique
Tien-tu	In the depression above the suprasternal notch.
	Lie or sit down.
	Use index finger to press inward, then massage downward.

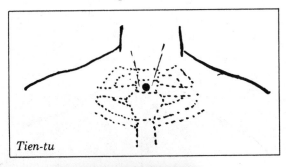

Tien-tu

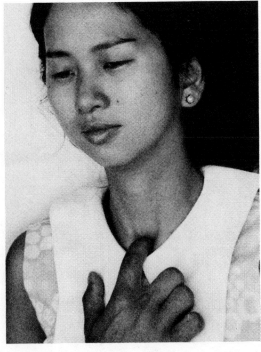

天突

Point	Location & Technique
Chuan-hsi	About 1 inch lateral to the lower end of the 7th cervical disk.
	Sit down and bend the head forward.
	Use thumb to massage hard toward the disk.

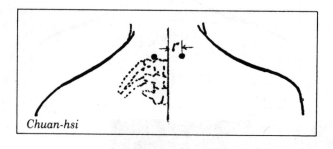

Chuan-hsi

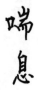

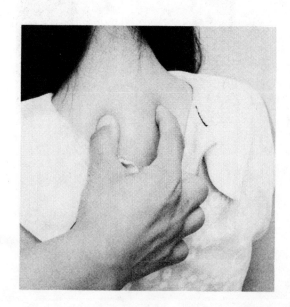

14

Point	Location & Technique
Fei-shu	About 1.5 inches lateral to the lower end of the 3rd thoracic disk.

Sit down or lie down on the stomach.

Use thumb to massage hard toward the disk.

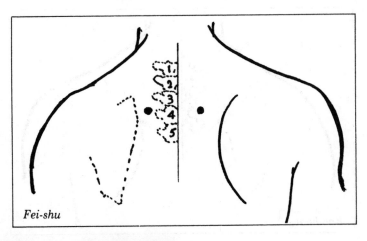

Fei-shu

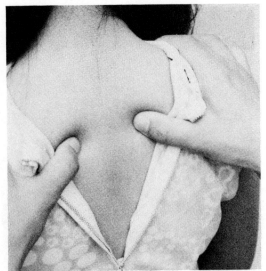

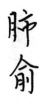

Point	Location & Technique
Kao-huang	About 3 inches lateral to the lower end of the 4th thoracic disk.

Sit down or lie down on the stomach.

Use thumb to massage hard.

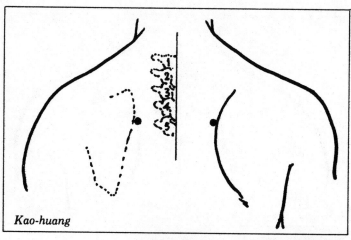

Kao-huang

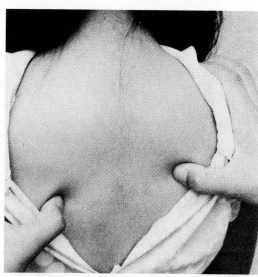

Point	Location & Technique
Nocturia	In the centers of the little finger creases.
	Lie or sit down.
	Use thumbnail to press hard. Try no. 1 first, if no result, try no. 1 and 2.

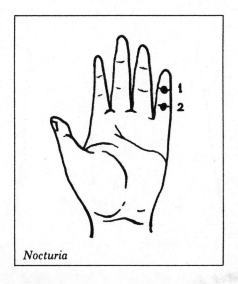

1
2

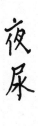

夜
尿

Nocturia

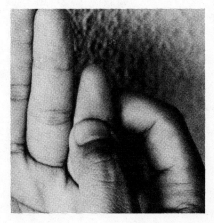
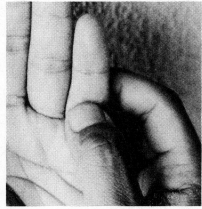

Point	Location & Technique
Chung-chi	About 4 inches below the navel, along the midline of the abdominal surface.
	Lie down.
	Use thumb or palm to press hard.

中
極

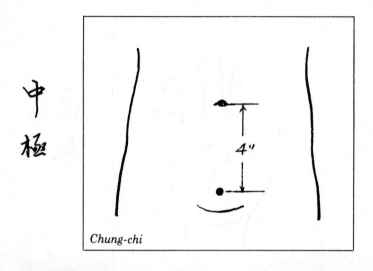

Chung-chi

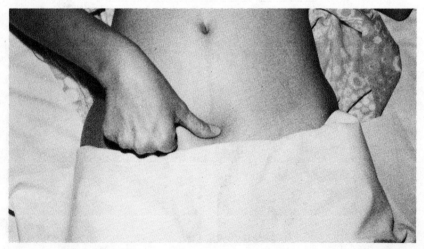

Point

Location & Technique

Chang-chiang

In between the tip of the tailbone and the anus.

Lie down on the stomach.

Use index finger to press downward, then massage upward.

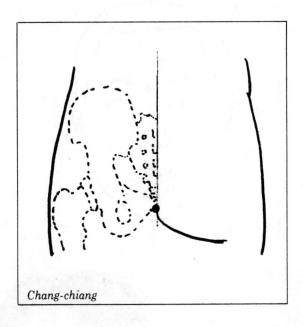

Chang-chiang

Point	Location & Technique
Yin-Tang	In between the eyebrows.
	Lie or sit down.
	Use thumb and index finger to pinch hard.

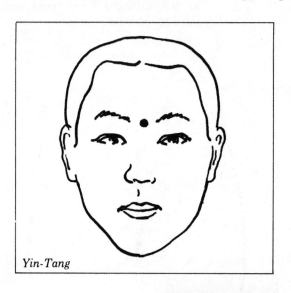

Yin-Tang

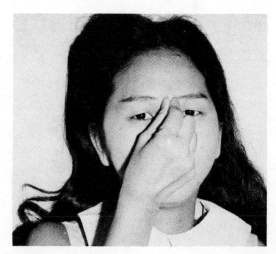

Point	Location & Technique
Tai-chung	Over the depression in between the 1st and 2nd metatarsal bones.

Lie or sit down.

Use thumbnail to press hard.

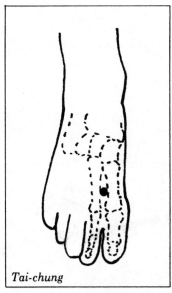

Tai-chung

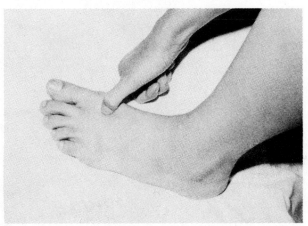

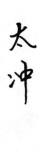

Point	Location & Technique
*Tongue-tip**	At the tip of the tongue.
	Any posture.
	Use front teeth to bite the tip of the tongue, and swallow the saliva.

*This is not an acupuncture point.

Point	**Location & Technique**
Chu-chih	At the external end of the elbow crease when the elbow is bent at 90°.

Lie or sit down.

Use thumb to press hard.

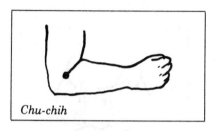

Chu-chih

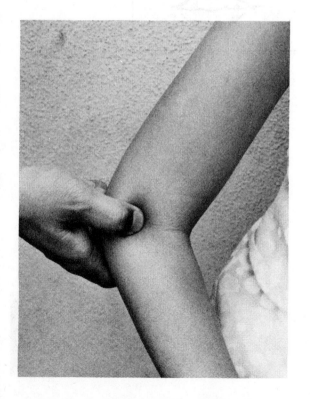

Point	Location & Technique
Jan-chung	Just above the middle of philtrum.
	Lie or sit down.
	Use thumbnail or index fingernail to press hard.

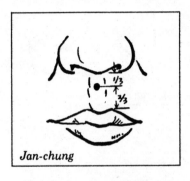

Jan-chung

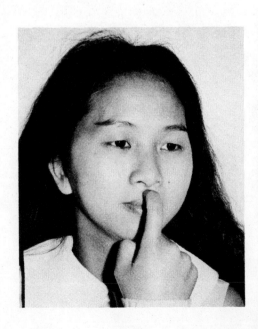

Point	Location & Technique
Yung-chuan	At the anterior one-third of the sole, between the 2nd and 3rd metatarsal bones.

Lie down.
Use thumbnail to press hard.

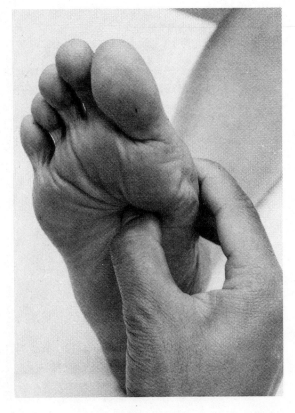

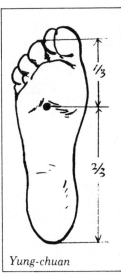

Yung-chuan

Frontal, vertical, occipital, and migraine.

Point	Location & Technique
Ho-ku	Over the dorsum of the hand, in between the 1st and 2nd metacarpal bones.
	Lie or sit down.
	Use thumb to press against the 2nd metacarpal bone.

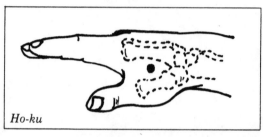

Ho-ku

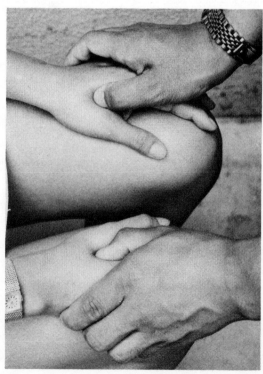

Point

Feng-chih

Location & Technique

Below the occipital bone, about 1.5 inches lateral to the midline of the head.

Sit down and bend the head forward.

Use thumb to massage hard.

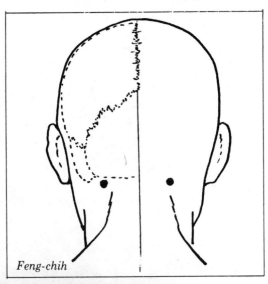

Feng-chih

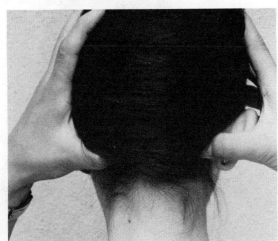

Point

Jan-chung

Location & Technique

Just above the middle of philtrum.

Lie or sit down.

Use thumbnail or index fingernail to press hard.

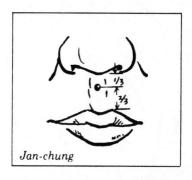

Jan-chung

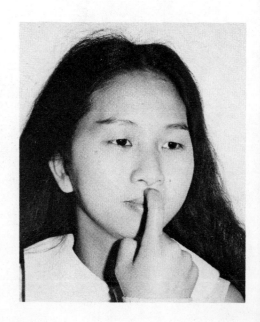

Point	Location & Technique
Yung-chuan	At the anterior one-third of the sole, between the 2nd and 3rd metatarsal bones. Lie down. Use thumbnail to press hard.

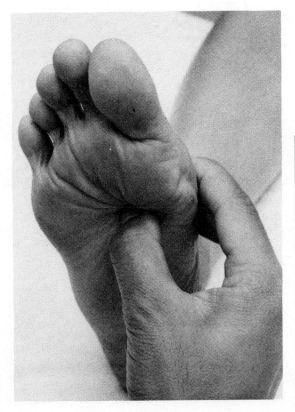

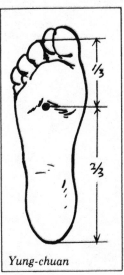

Yung-chuan

29

Point	Location & Technique
Hysteria	At the center of the bottom crease of the thumb.
	Any posture.
	Use thumbnail to press hard.

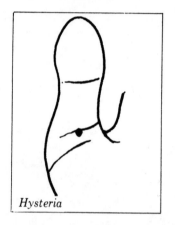

Hysteria

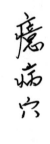

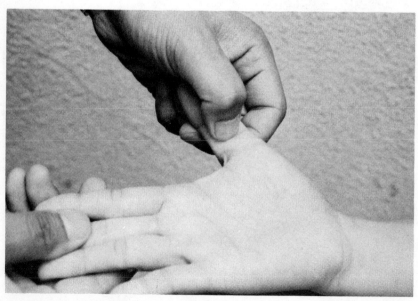

Early ejaculation

Point	Location & Technique
*Penis**	At the tip of the penis. Any posture. Use thumb and index finger to squeeze the tip of the penis, while the penis is still erecting before orgasm.

*This is not an acupuncture point. Needle insertion is prohibited.

No erection

Point	Location & Technique
Kuan-yuan	About 3 inches below the navel, along the midline of the abdominal surface.

Lie down.

Use thumb or palm to massage hard.

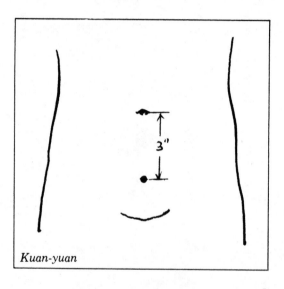

Kuan-yuan

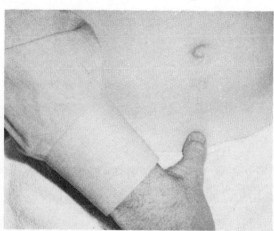

No erection

Location & Technique

San-yin-chiao   About 3 inches above the medial ankle, behind the tibia.

Lie down.

Use thumb to press hard.

三
阴
交

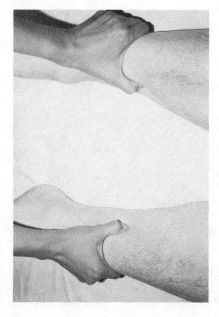

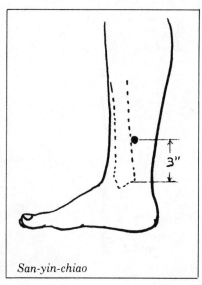

San-yin-chiao

No erection

Point	Location & Technique
Tsu-san-li	About 3 inches below the kneecap, 1 inch lateral to the tibia.

Lie down.

Use thumb to press down, then massage upward.

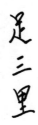

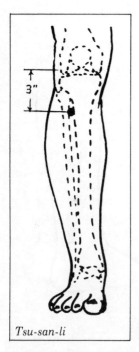

Tsu-san-li

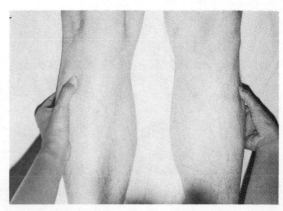

No erection

Point	Location & Technique

Shen-shu

About 1.5 inches lateral to the lower end of the 2nd lumbar disk.

Lie down on the stomach.

Use thumb to press hard toward the spine

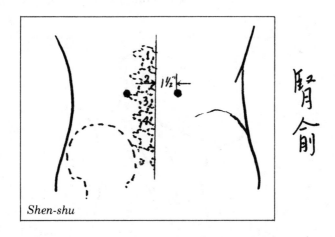

Shen-shu

腎
俞

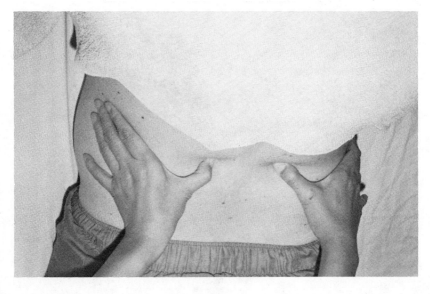

Point	Location & Technique
An-mien	About 1 inch behind the lobule of the ear.
	Lie or sit down.
	Use index finger to press hard.

If this point does not work, see page 37.

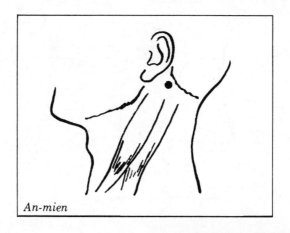

An-mien

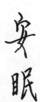

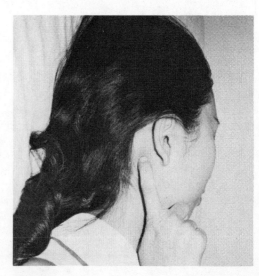

Point	Location & Technique
Shen-man	Along the most distal skin crease of the wrist, on the ulnar side, medial to the tendon. Lie or sit down. Use thumbnail to press hard.

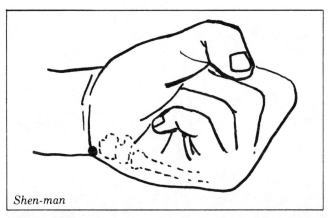

Shen-man

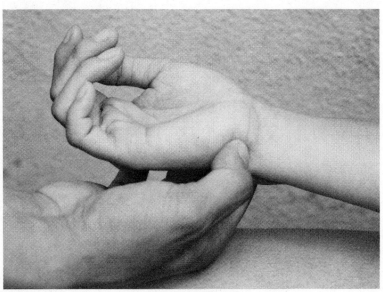

Point	Location & Technique
San-yin-chiao	About 3 inches above the medial ankle, behind the tibia.
	Lie or sit down.
	Use thumb to press hard.

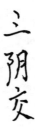

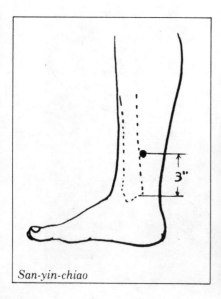

San-yin-chiao

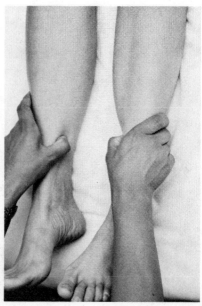

Point	**Location & Technique**
Chi-yen	In the two depressions below the kneecap.
	Sit down and bend the knee.
	Use thumb and index finger to press hard at the two depressions at the same time.

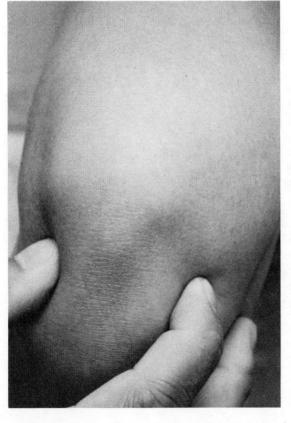

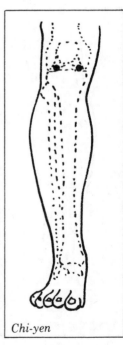

Chi-yen

39

Point

Yang-ling-chuan

Location & Technique

About 2 inches below the kneecap, just in front of fibula.

Sit down and bend the knee.

Use thumb to press hard.

阳
陵
泉

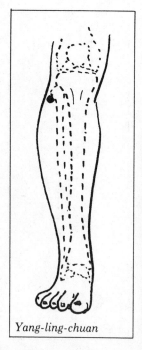

Yang-ling-chuan

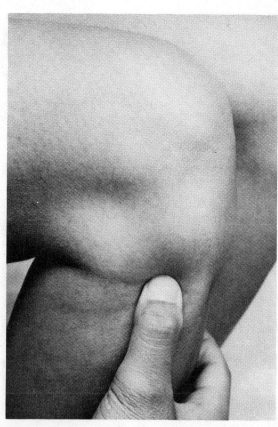

Point	Location & Technique

Chia-che

Over the masseteric muscle.

Sit or lie down.

Use both thumbs to massage both points at the same time.

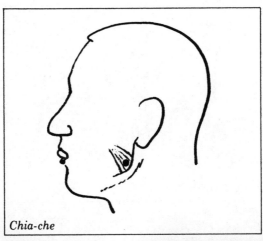

Chia-che

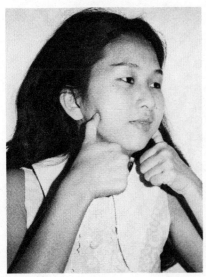
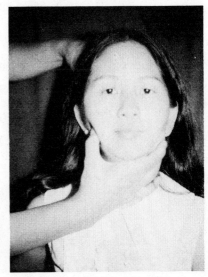

Point	Location & Technique
Shen-shu	About 1.5 inches lateral to the lower end of the 2nd lumbar disk.

Lie down on the stomach.

Use thumb to press hard toward the spine.

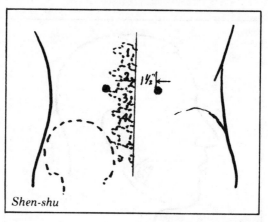

Shen-shu

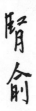

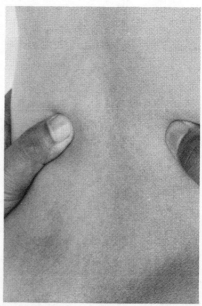

42

Nervousness

Point	Location & Technique
Shen-man 	Along the most distal skin crease of the wrist, on the ulnar side, medial to the tendon. Lie or sit down. Use thumbnail to press hard.

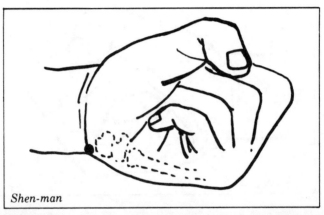

Shen-man

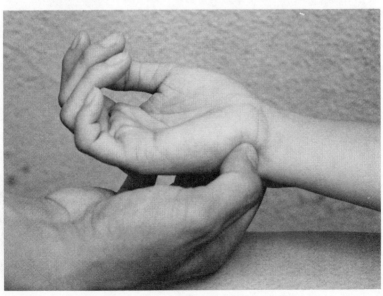

Point	Location & Technique

Point

Shen-man

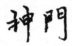

Location & Technique

Along the most distal skin crease of the wrist, on the ulnar side, medial to the tendon.

Lie or sit down.

Use thumbnail to press hard.

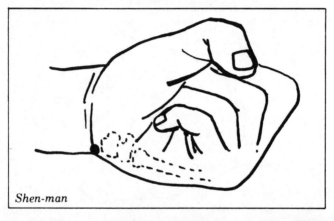

Shen-man

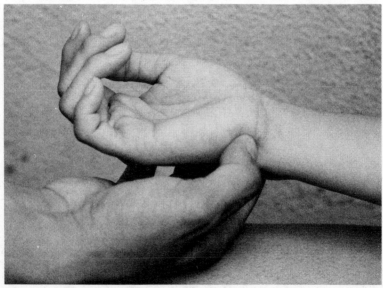

Point	Location & Technique
Tien-tu	In the depression above the suprasternal notch.

Lie or sit down.

Use index finger to press inward, then massage downward. |

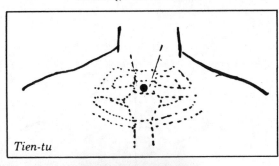

Tien-tu

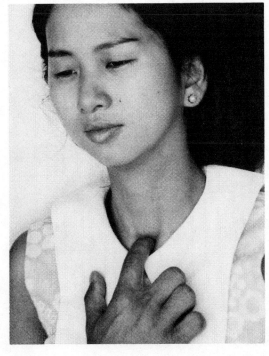

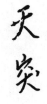

45

Point	Location & Technique

Point
Location & Technique

Chuan-hsi

About 1 inch lateral to the lower end of the 7th cervical disk.

Sit down and bend the head forward.

Use thumb to massage hard toward the disk.

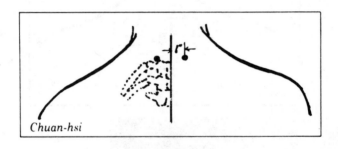

Chuan-hsi

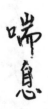

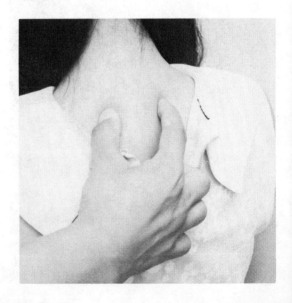

Point

Location & Technique

Fei-shu

About 1.5 inches lateral to the lower end of the 3rd thoracic disk.

Sit down or lie down on the stomach.

Use thumb to massage hard toward the disk.

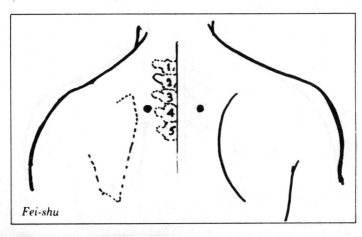

Fei-shu

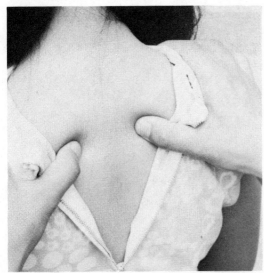

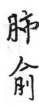

47

Point	**Location & Technique**
Kao-huang	About 3 inches lateral to the lower end of the 4th thoracic disk.
	Sit down or lie down on the stomach.
	Use thumb to massage hard.

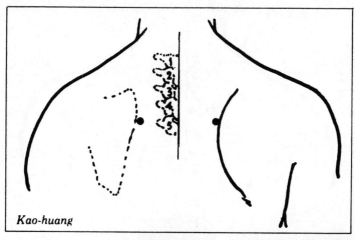

Kao-huang

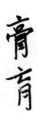

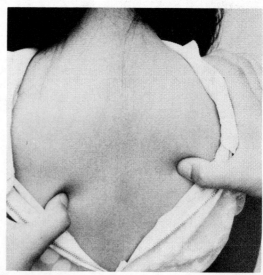

Point

Chien-yu

Location & Technique

At the antero-inferior part of the shoulder.

Sit down.

Use thumb to press hard.

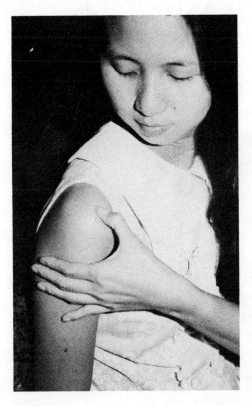

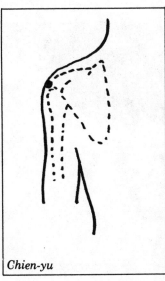

Chien-yu

Point

Chien-chin

Location & Technique

On the hump of the shoulder, along the same vertical line with the nipple.

Sit down.

Use thumb over Chien-chin and the other fingers over shoulder to squeeze and release. Repeat this action for about one minute.

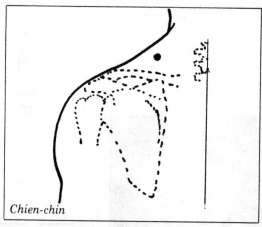

Chien-chin

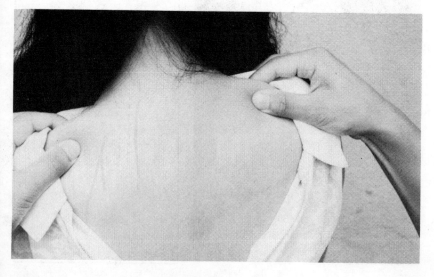

Point	Location & Technique
Yin-Tang	In between the eyebrows. Lie or sit down. Use thumb and index finger to pinch hard.

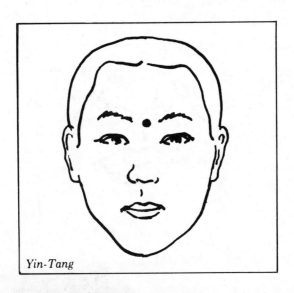

Yin-Tang

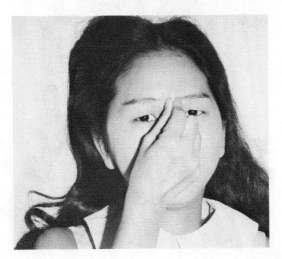

Point

Ying-hsiang

Location & Technique

By the side of the nose.

Lie or sit down.

Use index finger to massage.

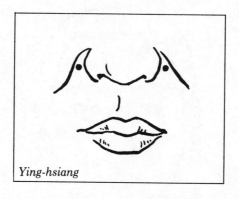

Ying-hsiang

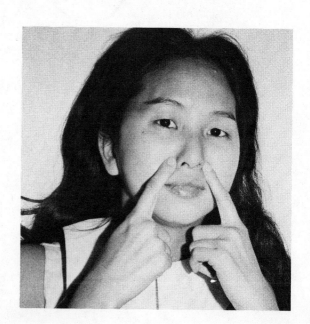

Point	Location & Technique
Shao-shang	About 0.1 inch away from the corner of thumbnail.
	Any posture.
	Use thumbnail to press hard.

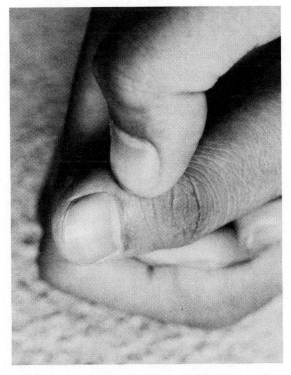

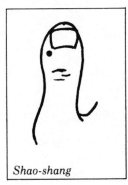

Shao-shang

Point	Location & Technique
Ho-ku	Over the dorsum of the hand, in between the 1st and 2nd metacarpal bone.

Any posture.

Use thumb to press hard against the 2nd metacarpal bone.

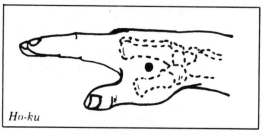

Ho-ku

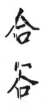

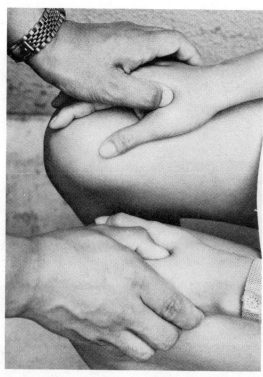

Point	Location & Technique
Feng-chih	Below the occipital bone, about 1.5 inches lateral to the midline of the head.

Sit down and bend the head forward.

Use thumb to massage hard.

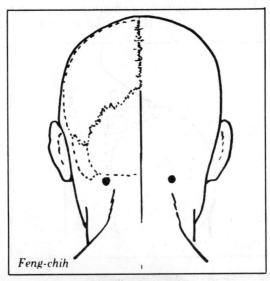

Feng-chih

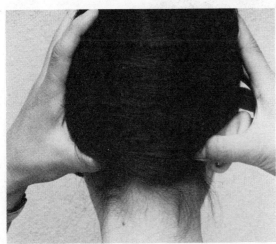

Point

Chien-chin

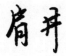

Location & Technique

On the hump of the shoulder, along the same vertical line with the nipple.

Sit down.

Use thumb over Chien-chin and the other fingers over shoulder to squeeze and release. Repeat this action for about one minute.

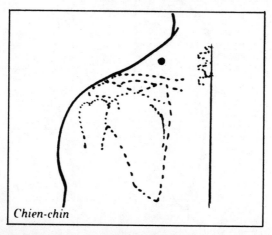

Chien-chin

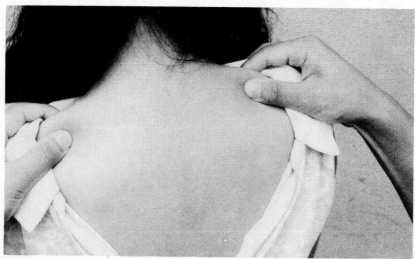

Point	Location & Technique
Jan-chung	Just above the middle of philtrum.
	Lie or sit down.
	Use thumbnail or index fingernail to press hard.

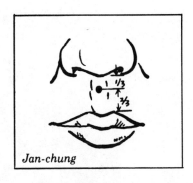

Jan-chung

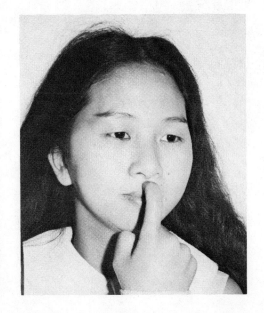

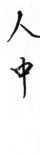

Point

Location & Technique

Yung-chuan

At the anterior one-third of the sole, between the 2nd and 3rd metatarsal bones.

Lie down.

Use thumbnail to press hard.

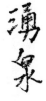

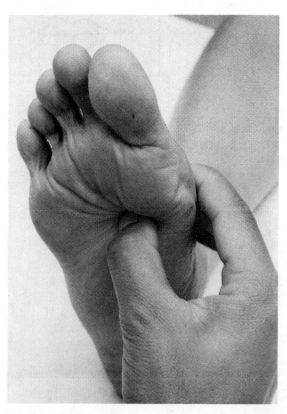

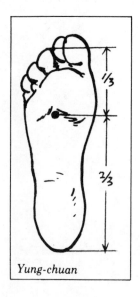

Yung-chuan

Point	Location & Technique
Polyhidrosis	At the center of the palm.
	Lie or sit down.
	Use thumbnail to press hard.

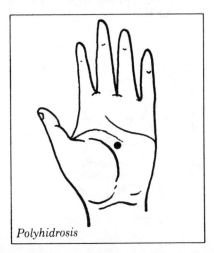

Polyhidrosis

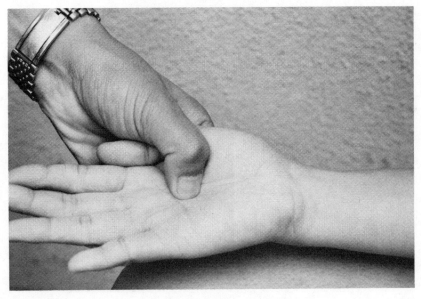

Point	Location & Technique
Jan-chung	Just above the middle of philtrum.
	Lie or sit down.
	Use thumbnail or index fingernail to press hard.

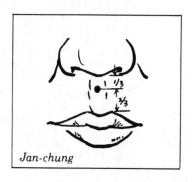

Jan-chung

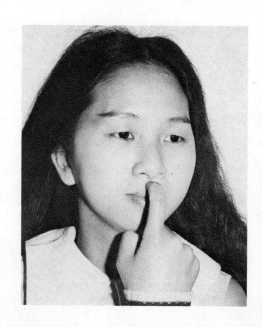

Point	Location & Technique
Yung-chuan	At the anterior one-third of the sole, between the 2nd and 3rd metatarsal bones.

Lie down.

Use thumbnail to press hard.

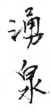

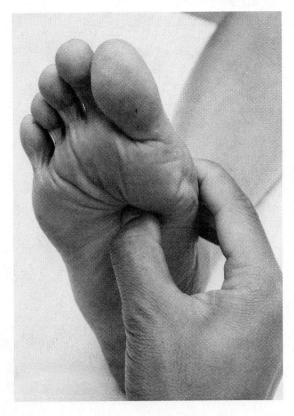

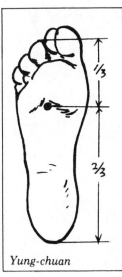

Yung-chuan

Upper jaw, lower jaw, or both

Point	Location & Technique
Ho-ku	Over the dorsum of the hand, in between the 1st and 2nd metacarpal bone.

Lie or sit down.

Use thumb to press against the 2nd metacarpal bone.

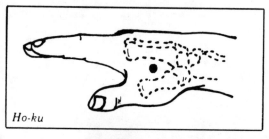

Ho-ku

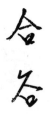

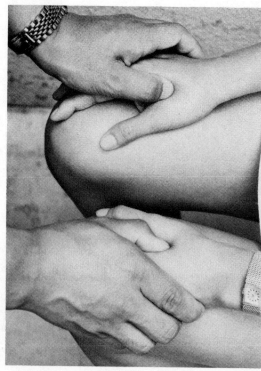

Upper jaw

Point	**Location & Technique**
Hsia-kuan	In the depression about 1 inch in front of the tragus.
	Lie or sit down.
	Use thumb to press hard.

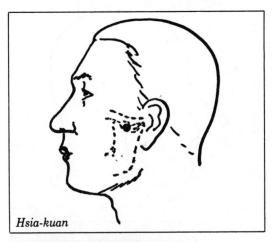

Hsia-kuan

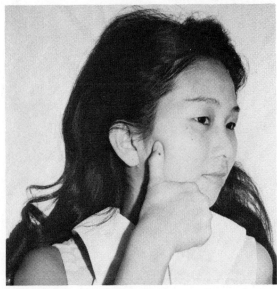

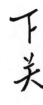

Lower jaw

Point	Location & Technique
Chia-che	Over the masseteric muscle. Sit or lie down. Use thumb to massage hard.

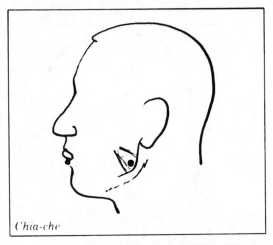

Chia-che

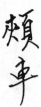

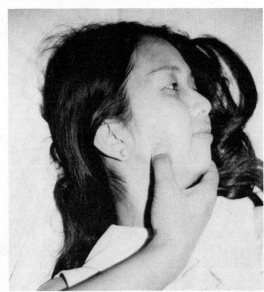

Point	Location & Technique
Tongue-tip*	At the tip of the tongue.
	Any posture.
	Use front teeth to bite the tip of the tongue, and swallow the saliva.

* This is not an acupuncture point.

Point	Location & Technique
Ho-ku	Over the dorsum of the hand, in between the 1st and 2nd metacarpal bones.

Lie or sit down.

Use thumb to press against the 2nd metacarpal bone.

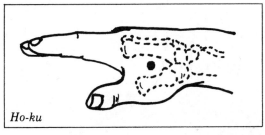

Ho-ku

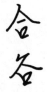

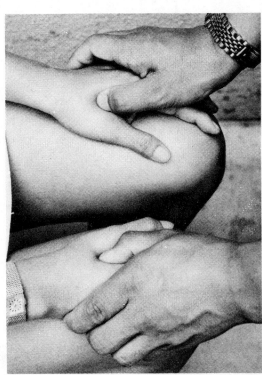

Point	Location & Technique
Kun-lun	In the depression behind the lateral ankle.
	Lie or sit down.
	Use thumb to press hard.

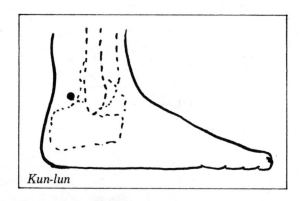

Kun-lun

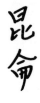

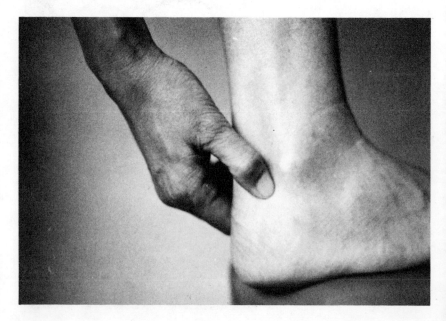

Point	Location & Technique
Ear Lobe	In the center of the ear lobe. Any posture. Put thumb and index fingers in between the ear lobe and press.

耳
垂

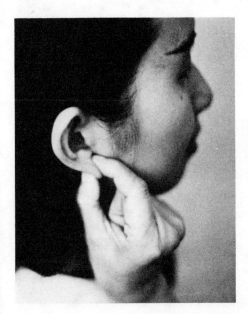

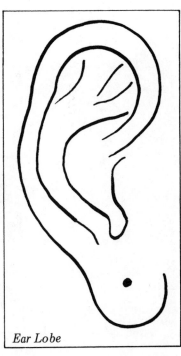

Ear Lobe

Point   **Location & Technique**

Over the dorsum of the hand, in between the 1st and 2nd metacarpal bones.

Lie or sit down.

Use thumb to press against the 2nd metacarpal bone.

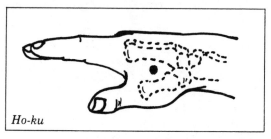

Ho-ku

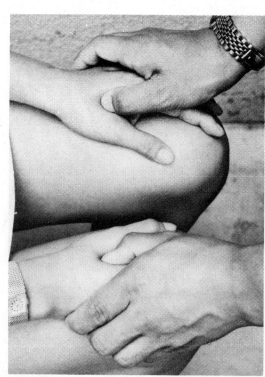

Point

Ta-chui

Location & Technique

In between the 7th cervical and the 1st thoracic vertebra.

Sit or lie down on one's side. The head should be bent down slightly.

Use the tip of the index finger to press and massage.

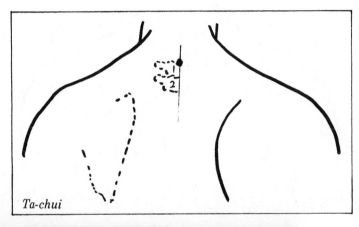

Ta-chui

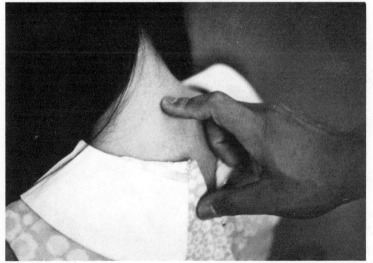

大椎

73

Point

Feng-men

Location & Technique

About 1.5 inches lateral to the lower
end of the spine of the second thoracic
vertebra.
Sit or lie down on one's side.
Use the thumb to massage.

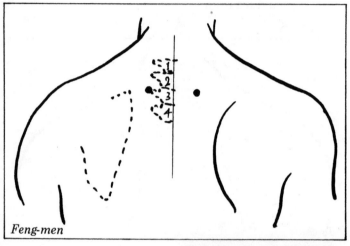

Feng-men

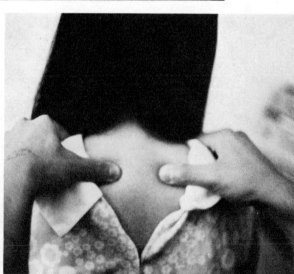

74

If with fever, add

Point   **Location & Technique**

Chu-chih

At the external end of the elbow crease when the elbow is bent at 90°.

Lie or sit down.

Use thumb to press hard.

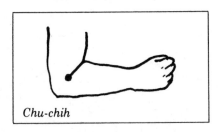

Chu-chih

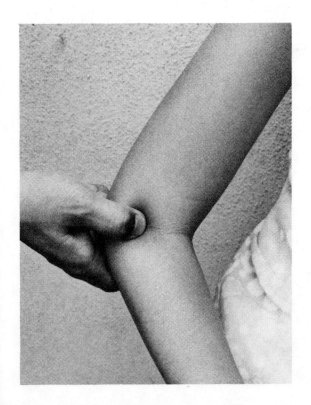

If with Cough, add

Point	Location & Technique
Tien-tu	In the depression above the suprasternal notch.
	Lie or sit down.
	Use index finger to press inward, then massage downward.

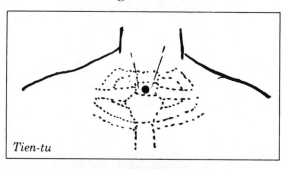

Tien-tu

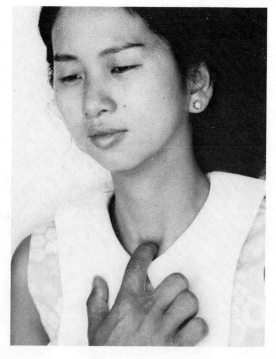

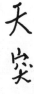

Point	**Location & Technique**
San-yin-chiao	About 3 inches above the medial ankle, behind the tibia.
	Lie or sit down.
	Use thumb to press hard.

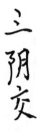

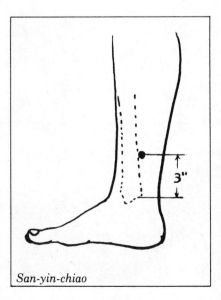

San-yin-chiao

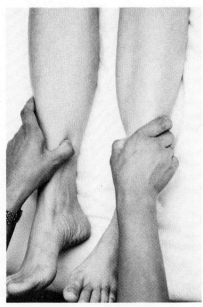

Point	Location & Technique
Chih-yin	About one-tenth of an inch behind the lateral corner of the little toenail. Lie down. Use the thumbnail to press down.

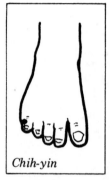

Chih-yin

至
陰

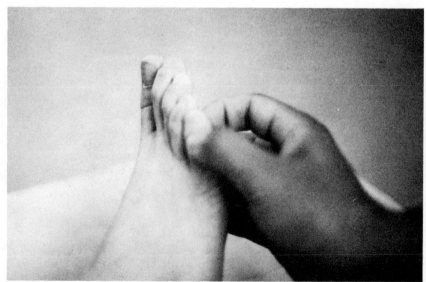

Point	Location & Technique
Vertex	On the radial side of the doral surface of the phalangeal joint of the middle finger. Any posture. Use the thumbnail to press hard.

頭
頂
点

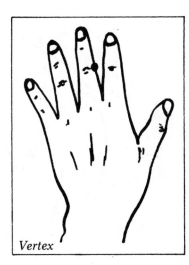

Vertex

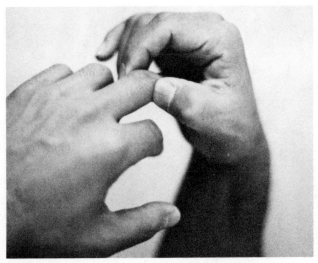

Point	Location & Technique
Ke-shu	About 1.5 inches lateral to the lower end of the 7th thoracic vertebra. Sit or lie down on one's side. Use thumb to press down and hard.

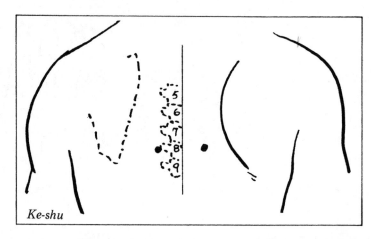

膈
俞

Ke-shu

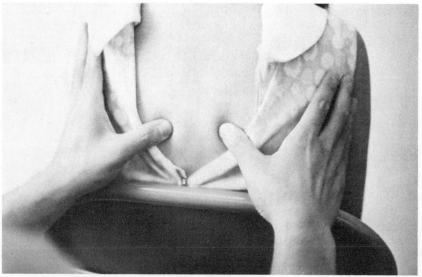

Point	Location & Technique
Jen-ying	By side of Adam's Apple.

Use two fingers to press down very lightly. Press and release. Be sure not to press hard.

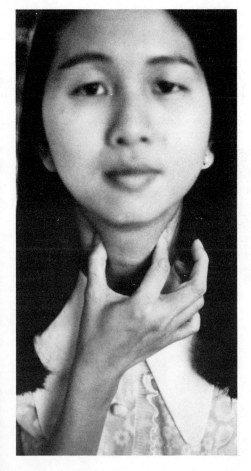

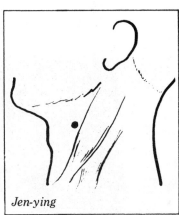

Jen-ying

Point   **Location & Technique**

Blood Pressure point About 2 inches lateral to the lower end
of the 6th cervical vertebra.

Sit or lie down on one's side.

Use thumbs to press and massage both points.

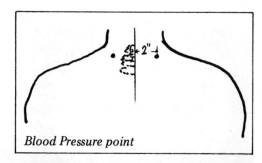

Blood Pressure point

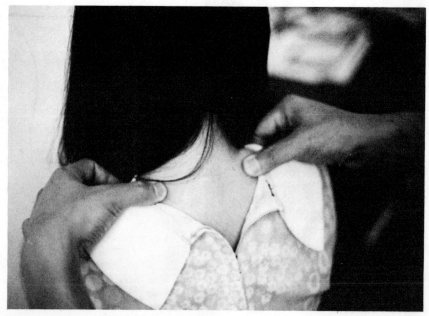

Point	Location & Technique
Depressing Groove	A curved vertical groove on the back of the ear. Any posture. Use fingernail to press down and hard.

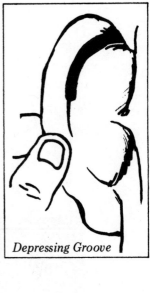

Depressing Groove

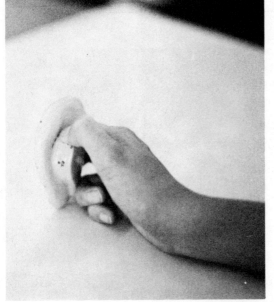

降压沟

Point	Location & Technique
An-mien	About 1 inch behind the lobule of the ear.
	Lie or sit down.
	Use index finger to press hard.

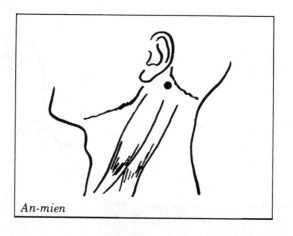

An-mien

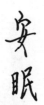

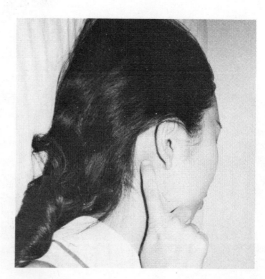

Point	Location & Technique
Nei-kuan	About 2 inches above the middle of the palmar wrist crease, in between the two tendons.

Any posture.

Use the tip of the finger to press down and massage.

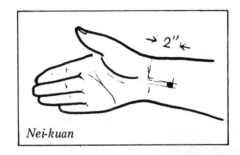

Nei-kuan

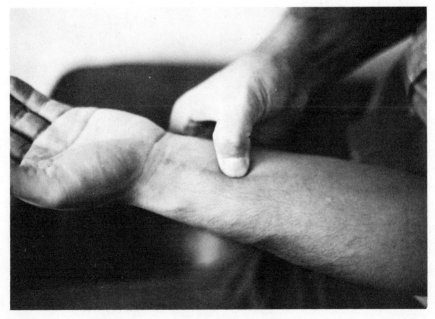

Point	Location & Technique
Tsu-san-li	About 3 inches below the kneecap, 1 inch lateral to the tibia.

Lie down.

Use thumb to press down, then massage upward.

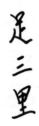

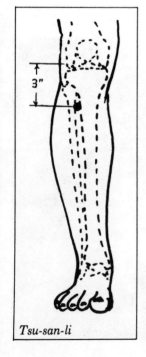

Tsu-san-li

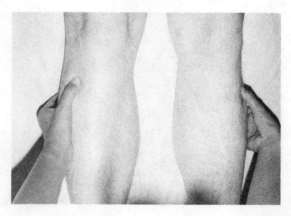

Point	**Location & Technique**
San-yin-chiao	About 3 inches above the medial ankle, behind the tibia.
	Lie or sit down.
	Use thumb to press hard.

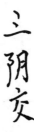

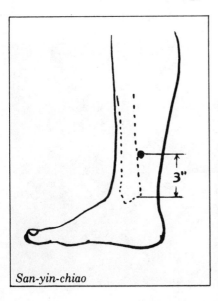

San-yin-chiao

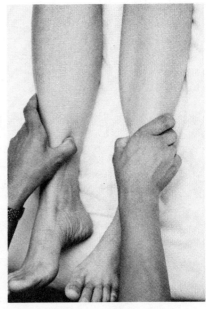

Point	**Location & Technique**
Szu-feng	On the palmar surface, middle of the proximal joint crease of the second, middle, fourth and the little finger.
	Any posture.
	Use the fingernail to press down.

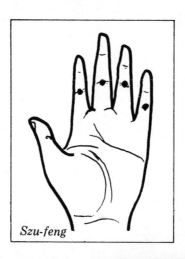

Szu-feng

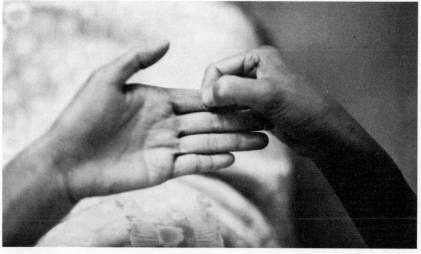

Point	Location & Technique
Yang-lao	Along the seam on the radial side of the distal head of the ulna.
	Any posture.
	Use fingernail to press down and hard.

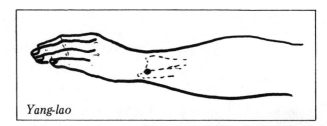

Yang-lao

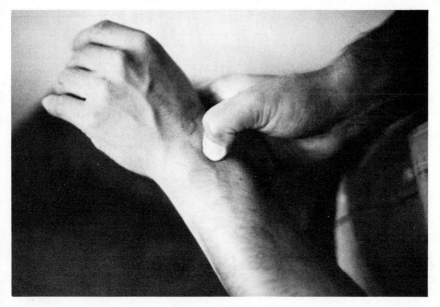

Chinese name		English equivalent	Meridian	Page
Feng-men	風府	Wind gate	Bladder 12	74
Ho-ku	合谷	Meeting valley	Large intestine 4	26, 54, 62, 69, 72
Hsia-kuan	下关	Low gate	Stomach 7	63
Hysteria	癔病	Hysteria	New point	30
Jan-chung	人中	Man center	Governing 26	24, 28, 57, 60
Jen-ying	人迎	Men welcome	Stomach 9	81
Kao-huang	膏肓	Vital organ	Bladder 38	16, 48
Ke-shu	膈俞	Diaphragm point	Bladder 17	80
Kuan-yuan	关元	Closing origin	Conception 4	32
Kun-lun	昆仑	Mountain	Bladder 60	70
Nei-kuan	内关	Inner gate	Pericardium 6	85
Nocturia	夜尿	Nocturia	New point	17
Polyhidrosis	多汗	Polyhidrosis	New point	59
San-yin-chiao	三阴交	3 females meeting	Spleen 6	33, 38, 77, 87
Shao-shang	少商	Young merchant	Lung 11	53
Shen-man	神門	Divine gate	Heart 7	37, 43, 44

91

Chinese name		English equivalent	Meridian	Page
Shen-shu	腎俞	Kidney point	Bladder 23	35
Szu-feng	四縫	Four sewing	Non-meridian point	88
Ta-chui	大椎	Big hammer	Governing 14	73
Tai-chung	太冲	Too rushy	Liver 3	21, 42
Tien-tu	天突	Sky prominence	Conception 22	13, 45, 76
Tsu-san-li	足三里	Foot 3 miles	Stomach 36	11, 34, 86
Vertex	頭頂尖	Vertex	New point	79
Yang-Lao	養老	Feeding the old	Small intestine 6	89
Yang-ling chuan	陽陵泉	Yang mound spring	Gall bladder 34	40
Ying-hsiang	迎香	Welcome fragrance	Large intestine 20	52
Yin-tang	印堂	Stamp hall	Non-meridian point	20, 51
Yung-chuan	湧泉	Jumping spring	Kidney 1	29, 25, 58, 61

PRICE/STERN/SLOAN
Publishers, Inc., Los Angeles